An Easy Way To Understand Parasites, Worms, Candida, Constipation & Detoxing

Brian B Jacques.

Part of a Series of Mini Health Books

Wisdom For Life Media

Copyright © 2014 Brian B Jacques. All rights reserved.

No part of this publication may be reproduced or transmitted in any form or by any means, mechanical or electronic, including photocopying and recording, or by any information storage and retrieval system without written permission from the publisher.

Publisher: Wisdom For Life Media

While they have made every effort to verify the information provided in this book, neither the author nor the publisher assumes any responsibility for errors in, omissions from, or different interpretation of the subject matter.

The information herein may be subject to varying laws, regulations, and practices in different areas, states and countries. The purchaser or reader assumes all responsibility for use of the information.

All information included within this book is for educational purposes only. The author and publishers do not attempt to diagnose or treat any medical conditions, be it to do with health, diet or exercise.

If you consider that you have any kind of medical condition, then, you should consult a qualified medical practitioner or doctor before starting any vitamin and/or mineral program or supplement regime, exercise or health training program or diet suggested in this book.

This book is not intended for anyone under the age of 18 years, nor is it intended for breast feeding or pregnant women, underweight people or anyone with eating disorders or a health condition that requires special diets or medical treatment.

The author and publishers disclaim any liability for any loss however caused by anyone using the information contained in this book.

ISBN - 13: 978-1499717068

Contents

Parasites—An Invisible Attack 7

Human Parasites 8

So Where Do They Come From? 9

Types Of Parasites 10

  Worms 10

    Pinworms   10
    Hookworms   10
    Roundworms   11
    Tapeworms   11
    Liver fluke   11

  Protozoa 11

    Giardia lamblia 11
    Entamoeba histolytica 12
    Cryptosporidium   12
    Toxoplasma gondii   12

Destination Diagnosis - Yet More Symptoms 13

Can There Be Complications? 14

How Do I Stop Myself Getting Infected With Parasites? 15

Some Dietary Guidelines To Prevent Parasites 17

Drug Treatment & Cure 18

    Albendazole   18
    Furazolidone   18
    Iodoquinol   18
    Mebendazole   18
    Metrodidazole 18
    Niclosamide   18
    Paromomycin 18
    Pyrantel pamoate 19
    Pyrimethamine 19
    Quinacrine   19
    Sulfadiazine   19
    Thiabendazole 19

Alternative Methods 20

Herbal Products For Parasites 20

    Black Walnut 20
    Cloves 20
    Colloidal Silver 20
    Grapefruit Seed Extract 20
    Garlic 20
    Pumpkin Seeds 21

Then Along Came Candida 22

The Symptoms 23

Treatment 24

Drug Treatment And Cure 24

    Diflucan 24
    Nystatin 24
    Sporanox 24
    Nizoral (ketoconazole) 24

Alternative Methods 25

Herbal Products For Candida 26

    Acidophilus 26
    Antioxidants 26
    Apple Cider Vinegar 26
    Natural Multi Vitamin & Multi Mineral Supplement 26
    Caprylic Acid 26
    Colloidal Silver 26
    Flaxseed Oil 26
    Garlic 27
    Grapefruit Seed Extract 27
    Oregano 27
    Pau D' Arco 27
    Peppermint Oil 28
    Probiotics 28

Constipation 29

What Can I Do? 29

Herbal Products For Constipation 30

    Cascara Sagrada 30
    Guar Gum 30
    Psyllium 30

Detoxing With A Herbal Colon Cleanse 31

Herbal Products For Detoxing 34

Diuretic and Laxative Herbs 34

    Alfalfa 34
    Cascara Sagrada 34
    Guar Gum 34
    Hibiscus Flower 34
    Licorice Root 34
    Marshmallow Root 35
    Psyllium 35
    Violet Leaf 35
    Yucca Root 35

Liver Support Herbs 36

    Cascara Sagrada 36
    Dandelion 36
    Milk Thistle 36

Parasite Expulsion Herbs 36

    Black Walnut 36
    Garlic 36
    Pumpkin Seeds 37

Herbs to Soothe an Irritated Digestive System & Urinary Tract 37

    Cranberry 37
    Irish Moss 37
    Passionflower 37

Herbs that have Antioxidant, Antiseptic and Anti-Inflammatory Properties 37

    Capsicum 37
    Chickweed 38
    Cranberry 38
    Gentian Root 38
    Witch Hazel 38

Herbs that Act as Blood Purifiers, Diuretics and Energy Providers 38

- Burdock Root 38
- Chlorella 38
- Echinacea 39
- Fennel Seed 39
- Fenugreek 39
- Garlic 39
- Ginger 39
- Horsetail 40
- Mullein 40
- Oatstraw 40
- Slippery Elm 40

Skin Cleansing Herbs 40

- Burdock Root 40
- Capsicum 40
- Colloidal Silver 41
- Ginger 41
- Oregano 41
- Peppermint Oil 41
- Yellow Dock 41

To Sum Up 42

Notice To My Readers 44

About The Author 45

Parasites—An Invisible Attack

We're under siege. All around us are small creatures which want to attack every cell in our bodies. But the problem is we can't even see them so most of us assume they are not even there.

It might sound like something from a sci-fi movie but we're constantly under invasion – from various parasites, protozoa, amoeba, bacteria and fungi. These aren't just germs but organisms which find their way into our bodies and make their homes there. Sounds scary? Well, don't worry. We have ways of eradicating them.

Parasites lurk everywhere in our environment. It's very easy indeed to get infected by them. It's a question of knowing what to do when they make it into your body.

Human Parasites

Whether we like it or not we play host to millions of unwelcome visitors in the form of human parasites which invade our bodies and make it their home. Since these tiny creatures have no way of making food for themselves, they rely on us instead for their day to day survival.

And by the way there are a hundred separate parasites which can invade and attack the human body.

But like all parasites, ultimately, they damage their hosts. We're damaged because they're busy stealing our food and nutrients. Not only that. They're busy destroying our tissue and cells in the process. They produce poisonous waste which can make us very ill and in some cases even kill us.

Another thing to remember. These invisible invaders well deserve the title of "prolific". They can hatch literally tens of thousands of eggs at a time.

It's a huge problem especially in less developed countries, but the USA and Europe are not immune to these problems either. In some Third World countries human parasite infections have reached alarming and epidemic proportions. They're claiming the lives of many thousands of people. Even more are being made dangerously ill by these things. Even in the world's richest country, the United States, things are getting out of hand. The figures are quite shocking.

According to experts, half the population of the United States have some kind of parasite infection.

Admittedly only about a quarter of these have active parasitic infections which show any symptoms. Nevertheless, the situation's getting worrying—and you need to be made aware of the problem, and in this book I offer some solutions for you to consider.

So Where Do They Come From?

Given the fact that we're a global village these days with millions of people constantly flying across continents, in many ways it's not really surprising. Over the past few decades we've seen tens of millions of people uproot themselves and move to the US and Europe especially. Often they bring parasites with them—as do military personnel returning from conflict zones overseas.

In many developed countries–despite all the precautions–many young children pick up parasites from day care centers. Even our pets also pose a big threat. Huge numbers of people pick up parasites from their cats and dogs. It seems you can't escape. Going out to restaurants for meals can leave you more vulnerable than those who eat at home. Why? Because restaurant staff handling food are known to spread parasites—not deliberately, of course.

Some people are more likely to pick up parasites than others. People living in warm, humid areas have a greater risk. So do people in such jobs as animal handlers, plumbers, electricians, gardeners and sanitation workers as well as those who regularly travel abroad.

We can pick up parasites from all sorts of different places:

- Insect bites
- Animal feces
- Walking barefoot
- Handling raw meat and fish
- Eating raw or undercooked pork, beef or fish
- Handling soiled litter pans (cats)
- Eating contaminated raw fruits and vegetables
- Eating meals prepared by infected food handlers
- Drinking contaminated water
- Having contact with infected persons (including sexual contact, kissing, and shaking hands)
- Inhaling contaminated dust (parasitic eggs or cysts)

That's quite a long list. It seems like there's no escape, doesn't it?

Types Of Parasites

We're going to look in more detail now at this small-scale but devastating enemy and work out an order of battle.

First we need to understand exactly what they are, how they enter our body and what they do. Some parasites are tiny amoeba and protozoa which are so small you can only see them through a microscope. Others such as worms and flukes are much larger. But whatever their size, they still cause problems.

We normally only get infected by worms when we eat infected meat, fish or from our pets.

It's the amoeba and protozoa which pose the greatest degree of risk to us. They reach us through the air, via water, food, animals, insects and even human contact. They travel from our intestines and into our bloodstream, vital organs and muscles. Once lodged in these places they're free to cause maximum damage and often this can be considerable. They can be extremely infectious.

They've been linked to cancer, rheumatoid arthritis, asthma, diabetes, multiple sclerosis, pyorrhoea (a deterioration of the gums and the tissues surrounding your teeth) and other diseases.

Let's have a look at the main types of parasites, beginning with the ones we can normally see.

Worms

Pinworms

This is one of the most common types of worm. Although this worm sets up home in your colon, it lays its eggs outside your body. It means that you can pick up pinworms through unclean hands or dirty clothes and bed linen. You'll know if you've got it by the irritation and itchiness in your anal area.

Hookworms

This one lives in your intestines where it firmly attaches itself and proceeds to start sucking your blood. But it actually starts life outside your body in soil or water and this is how you get infected. Sometimes we pick it up by drinking water contaminated with hookworm larvae. Or it may get into our bodies via fruit or vegetables. The symptoms of having hookworms are general weakness, nausea, abdominal pain, diarrhea and anemia.

Roundworms

These are one of the most common parasites in the world and can be as large as a pencil. We absorb them into our system by ingesting eggs found in soil, fruit and vegetables. They start off in the intestine but then move off to attack other organs where the can do severe damage. If you've suffered weight loss, feel weak, have infections or find yourself with abdominal pain you may be infected.

Tapeworms

These are more common in cats and dogs than in people. To get infected you'd have to swallow the fleas which are themselves infected with tapeworm larvae. Like its cousins it takes up residence in the intestines where it steals vital nutrients and then excretes toxic waste into your gut. The big snag we face here is that people with tapeworms often don't show any symptoms. When they do it shows up as mineral problems, feeling bloated, dizziness, hunger pains, digestive problems, sensitivity to touch, allergies and not being able to think straight. A tapeworm can live inside the body for 25 – 30 years.

Liver fluke

These are particularly unpleasant. They attack your liver by drilling holes into it and causing inflammation. And—wait for it—these flukes can survive in your body for up to 30 years! We get them by eating undercooked fish, contaminated vegetables or human feces when it's used as fertilizer. It can also be acquired by drinking or swimming in contaminated water. It causes an enlarged liver, pains on the right side of the body, depression, edema (a build up of fluid beneath the skin), vertigo, bile stones and in some cases cancer.

Protozoa

These come in a great many shapes and sizes but we'll focus on the four most common types.

Giardia lamblia

Apart from pinworm this is about the most common type of parasite that affects humans. It's very widespread. These microbes hide in your intestine or gall bladder. It's spread through fecal contamination as well as through water. But there are other risk factors such as dirty water or unsafe sexual practices. It's a bit of a tough guy this one and is resistant to chlorine, which means that you can still pick it up through tap water or from rivers and streams. Pains in your abdomen, sensitivity to food, diarrhea and vitamin deficiency are all symptoms.

Entamoeba histolytica

This is very tiny—just a single cell—but it causes a disease called amebiasis, an infection of the liver, intestines and other tissues. We find it in water and in damp places generally as well as in soil, vegetables and fruit. Again it can spread through fecal contamination, poor sanitation and unsafe sex as well as through crops fertilized by human waste. This is especially difficult because there aren't always symptoms, although in some warmer places it's the biggest killer after malaria. When symptoms do show up they appear as diarrhea, feelings of weakness, weight loss and pains in the abdomen.

Cryptosporidium

This one is often mentioned in the media especially when a hospital suffers an outbreak. It's another one-celled parasite which infects your digestive system and causes major gastro-intestinal upsets. Like the others this one is spread through feces via the mouth. It's widespread throughout the environment and it can infect public water supplies as well as rivers and lakes. It can also be spread through restaurants, day care centers and unsafe sex. Diarrhea, flu-like symptoms and pains in your stomach are the tell-tale signs you've got it.

Toxoplasma gondii

This is a crescent-shaped invader which attacks your central nervous system. It gets into our bodies by eating under-cooked meat or handling infected cat litter which can contain its eggs. The truth is that most of us have been exposed to this parasite at some time so we've built up defences in the form of antibodies to counteract it. Therefore, only a few people actually show up with symptoms which tend to be flu-like or you may experience fever, chills, tiredness and a headache.

Destination Diagnosis - **Yet More Symptoms**

Although we've talked a little bit about the symptoms already, these infections are often very tricky to diagnose because the symptoms are extremely vague—or in some cases there are absolutely no symptoms at all.

If you feel unwell, here are some indications that you may have an infestation:

- Diarrhea with foul-smelling stool that becomes worse in the later part of the day
- Sudden changes in bowel habits (e.g. constipation that is now a soft and watery stool)
- Constant rumbling and gurgling in the stomach area unrelated to hunger or eating
- Heartburn or chest pain
- Flu-like symptoms such as coughing, fever, and nasal congestion
- Food allergy
- Itching around the nose, ears, and anus, especially at night
- Loss of weight with constant hunger
- Anemia
- Anxiety caused by the metabolic waste products of the parasites

But even this isn't the end of the list because other symptoms could well include blood in the stool, bloating, diarrhea, gas, loss of appetite, intestinal obstruction and nausea. That's not to mention vomiting, sore mouth and gums, excessive nose picking, grinding teeth at night, chronic fatigue, headaches, muscle aches and pains, shortness of breath, skin rashes, depression and memory loss.

Normally these kinds of infections are diagnosed by simply looking at stool samples under a microscope. Usually one of the public health laboratories undertakes this work.

The big problem is that there's been a high failure rate in identifying just what's wrong. So sometimes blood tests are needed as well. But when you think there are dozens of different types of parasites, you'll understand that it's a big job identifying the correct ones.

Can There Be Complications?

Yes there can. But it's normally a problem that develops slowly. What happens is that worm populations build up over quite a long period of time. Eventually the health problems they cause get out of hand and become chronic.

For example, if you've got worms you might suffer from malnutrition because they steal nutrients from your body and deprive you of the benefits of the nutrients from your food. Or it may be that they simply reduce your appetite. Either way, you're not getting what you need to stay healthy. If you have parasites in your system over a long period of time it's likely to lead to food allergies.

Children who've got worms tend to be underweight and generally small for their age because worms have hampered their growth.

Roundworms can cause blockages in your colon. Intestinal worms, particularly hookworms can contribute to your having anemia because they cause loss of blood through bleeding in your intestines. The more worms you've got, the more problems you're likely to have.

Chronic parasite infections can be disastrous. They can stunt both your mental and physical development in the long term.

In some of the most severe cases they can even cause death.

How Do I Stop Myself Getting Infected With Parasites?

Like many other things in life, it's a question of common sense. Here's a quick list of some of the more obvious measures:

- Wash your hands before eating and after using the toilet.
- Wear gloves when you're gardening or working with soil or sand because these can be contaminated with eggs or cysts of parasites.
- Pregnant women should avoid handling cat litter.
- Don't allow children to be licked or kissed by pets that are not de-wormed regularly.
- Wear long-sleeved shirts, long pants, and boots especially when walking through tall grass or amongst trees. In addition, spray insect-repellent on clothing to prevent tick bites.
- Have a regular curry which is an effective antidote to parasites. You can follow this with a probiotic supplement which helps to cleanse your intestines.
- You could consider a regular colon cleanse.
- Always wash your hands, kitchen counters and utensils with hot soapy water after cutting or handling raw meat, chicken or fish.
- Don't use a microwave to cook meat, chicken or fish. Microwaves often don't heat foods completely.
- Always wear shoes or slippers (to prevent hookworm infection).
- Do not use water from septic tanks or other potentially contaminated sources for watering vegetables
- Contain all fecal matter (for example, by using a toilet or latrine, rather than "as nature intended" outside).
- Teach children proper hygiene i.e. washing hands after going to the toilet, playing outside and before preparing or eating food.
- If you have parasites, you can reduce the likelihood of passing them on to others by carefully washing your hands after having bowel movements and cleaning the genital area before having sex.

- Wear gloves when changing the cat box. Deworm pets periodically.
- Avoid swallowing river, stream or lake water when swimming in them. Better yet, avoid swimming in them altogether.
- Keep your body slightly acidic by including pumpkin seeds, calmyrna figs, garlic, apple cider vinegar, cranberry juice and pomegranates in your diet.
- Avoid eating water chestnuts and watercress.

Remember that you don't need to wander barefoot across a garbage dump to pick up parasites. They're everywhere. So beware.

If one member of the family is treated then all other members should be treated as well because there can easily be cross-infections or re-infections. Make sure everyone washes their hands frequently and that bed linen, clothes and even soft toys are kept clean.

Some Dietary Guidelines To Prevent Parasites

Eat as natural a diet as possible by buying organic meat, poultry, fruit and vegetables. Also include whole grains nuts and seeds. Make sure you get adequate fiber. Fiber assists in eradicating worms from the intestines; and a good nutrition regime supports the immune system which helps protect the body against parasitic infection.

- Parasites thrive on dairy foods, fats and sugar so use these sparingly.
- Avoid eating raw or under-cooked fish, pork or beef. Remember these foods are a breeding ground for fish tapeworm, pork tapeworm and beef tapeworm respectively.
- Supplement your diet with a high quality natural multi-vitamin and multi-mineral supplement to ensure you don't have a dietary shortfall in essential nutrients. If you diet is lacking, then the body will utilize what it needs from the supplement. If your body doesn't need it, then it will pass out in the urine.
- Make sure you have adequate "friendly" bacterial in your intestinal tract, especially if you have taken a course of antibiotics. Antibiotics not only kill harmful bacteria, but friendly bacteria too. A good probiotic supplement containing Lactobacillus acidophilus and other beneficial bacteria will ensure normal intestinal flora function which will help stop parasites from spreading.

Drug Treatment & Cure

The traditional way to treat parasites is by using a variety of drugs. This works on the basis of something we call "differential toxicity". All that means is that the drugs are more poisonous to the parasite than they are to you—hopefully. It doesn't always work out that way and there can be side-effects from these drugs such as nausea, abdominal pains, vomiting, headaches and rashes.

Depending on how severe your infection is you'll probably be provided with one of the following medications:

Albendazole

Albendazole is an anti-worm medication, and is used to treat certain infections caused by worms especially pork tapeworm and dog tapeworm. It prevents newly hatched insect larvae (worms) from growing or multiplying in the body.

Furazolidone

Furazolidone is taken by mouth and works in the intestinal tract. The drug is used to treat such conditions as cholera, colitis, and/or diarrhea caused by bacteria, giardiasis and protozoa. Protozoa are tiny, one-celled creatures some of which are parasites that if left untreated are the cause of many different kinds of infections in the body.

Iodoquinol

This medication is used to treat certain parasite infections in the intestines. It is either used alone or combined with other medications. It is not recommended to use this medication to treat a diarrhea condition where the cause is not determined.

Mebendazole

This medication is used to prevent worms such as hookworm, pinworm, roundworm and whipworm from growing and multiplying in the body.

Metrodidazole

This is an antibiotic which is used to treat a protozoa parasite infection.

Niclosamide

Niclosamide is used to treat various tape worm infestations such as beef tapeworm, dwarf tapeworm and fish tapeworm. It works by killing tapeworms on contact. The dead worms are then passed out in the feces. This medication will not work on other types of worms such as pinworms and roundworms.

Paromomycin

Paromomycin is an antibiotic which is used to treat various intestinal infections, as well as certain liver problems.

Pyrantel pamoate

This medication works by paralysing the nervous system of certain worms such as pinworm and roundworm which are then passed out in the feces.

Pyrimethamine

Pyrimethamine is used to prevent the growth and reproduction of parasites.

Quinacrine

Quinacrine is used in the treatment of the protozoa giardiasis in the intestinal tract.

Sulfadiazine

Sulfadiazine is an antibiotic, which is used to fight bacterial infections in the body.

Thiabendazole

Thiabendazole is a treatment used to prevent worms – such as threadworm from growing and multiplying in the body. In addition it may also be used to treat pinworm where this occurs with hookworm, roundworm, threadworm and whipworm.

Alternative Methods

Luckily, there are also much more gentle ways of dealing with lingering parasites such as herbal remedies, normally taken on an empty stomach before meals. You'll find a wide variety in shops and on the internet. I have included a list below.

Herbal Products For Parasites

Black Walnut

Black walnut is an excellent anti-parasitic herb, especially against worms. It also has a high iodine content, which is good for energy as it supports thyroid function.

Cloves

Cloves are a good natural parasite cleansing herb which can be obtained as a liquid, powder or in a capsule.

Colloidal Silver

Although not an herb, colloidal silver has many uses and has been found to be effective against many surface micro-organisms, viruses, protozoa, amoeba, fungi, parasites and yeasts.

There are many different colloidal silver products on the market. You need to source one that contains 99.9 percent pure silver, without any additives.

Grapefruit Seed Extract

Grapefruit seed extract is an effective anti-parasitic herb which has a very bitter taste. This can be sweetened by adding a small amount of honey.

Garlic

Garlic has so many uses from using it in cooking to it being an excellent product for heart health. It also has antibacterial, anti-fungus and antiviral properties. Other recognized health benefits of garlic, include acting as an antibiotic as well as other health advantages like its anti-cholesterol and anti-hypertensive properties.

It is also an antioxidant which protects the body against the effects of free radical damage. Its high sulphur content assists in cell purification.

Allicin is the principle biological active compound which gives garlic its odor. Be warned. Many so called "odourless" garlic products have the active compound removed which makes it rather worthless. It can be obtained as a garlic bulb, in a capsule or in tablet form.

Pumpkin Seeds

One of the best tasting of all the anti-parasite herbal products. The seeds can be eaten as a snack. In fact they taste so good that you cannot eat enough of them. Pumpkin seeds are very effective against tapeworms as well as other types of parasites. They also serve as a good source of essential fatty acids (EFAs) which are essential for good health.

Then Along Came Candida

Candida – or to give it its full name – Candidasis, is a yeast-like infection in your intestines. This is caused by an overgrowth of something called candida albicans. In many cases it can just be a bit of a nuisance but in other cases its effects can be far-reaching and very severe. We've seen an increase in these severe conditions recently. Many people make the mistake of thinking that it affects only women, but it affects men too.

What happens is that for some reason a normal single-celled organism suddenly starts behaving like a plant or tree and starts branching out into a fungal form known as mycelia. It produces long stem-like roots called rhizoids which break through the intestines and begin to invade other organs of the body. The candida alters the acidity of the intestine so that the healthy bacteria can't survive.

There's worse to come. The intestine walls are damaged and undigested proteins get into your blood and create a whole host of allergies and sensitivities. Like other fungi the candida produces an active substance known as mycotoxin (myco means fungus or mushroom). This can cause damage to the central nervous system and leave you with memory loss, confusion, fatigue, irritability, depressions, mood swings, headaches nausea, tingling, numbness and burning feelings. In fact it often leaves you feeling "sick all over".

One problem is that these systems are very reminiscent of many others and that makes candidasis hard to diagnose.

Another big snag is that once yeast has started blossoming it's very hard to eradicate. It's a disease that often becomes a vicious circle. For example, you've got a chest infection and so you start taking antibiotics.

Another problem is that antibiotics themselves prompt yeast overgrowth because they kill off healthy bacteria and throw the bacteria in the intestines completely off balance. The candida cells thrive and the result is a lowering of your immune system. This leads to you picking up further infections which are then treated with antibiotics again. And so on it goes, with little hope of ever eradicating the problem.

The Symptoms

Since candida leads to minerals and vitamins not being absorbed, you may have some of the following symptoms.

- Skin complaints.
- Poor appetite.
- Loss of sex drive.
- Muscle spasms or weakness.
- Poor memory.
- Insomnia.
- Depression.
- Confusion.
- Irregular heartbeat.
- Anemia.
- Reproductive problems.

Treatment

Realistically the medical treatments provided are likely to work best if you combine them with changes in your diet and modifications to your lifestyle to reduce stress and strengthen your immune system.

The most commonly prescribed medical candida remedies include anti-fungals which normally work within six to eight weeks.

The following is a brief list of medications.

Drug Treatment And Cure

Diflucan

Diflucan is an antifungal which is used to treat and prevent certain yeast and fungal infections. The mechanism it uses interferes with the formation of the fungal cell membrane.

Nystatin

Nystatin is an antifungal which is used in the treatment of fungal infections of the stomach, intestines, and mucous membranes. The mechanism it uses interferes with the formation of the fungal cell membrane, thus allowing the fungal cell contents to leak out and die.

Sporanox

Is an antifungal medication used to treat fungal infections which can invade any part of the body. For example: the mouth, throat, lungs, fingernails and toenails.

Nizoral (ketoconazole)

Nizoral (ketoconazole) is an antifungal antibiotic used to treat fungal infections which can invade any part of the body. For example: the mouth, throat, esophagus, lungs and skin.

Alternative Methods

The truth is that people often prefer more natural—or naturopathic—treatments. The main thing though is to cut out certain key things from your diet:

- Sugars
- Wheat and grain flours
- Sweet fruits
- Fermented foods or alcohol
- mushrooms
- Potatoes
- Yeast
- Corn
- Peanuts and cashew nuts
- Sausages, lunch meats and hotdogs
- Shellfish

Once you've climbed that mountain you need to eat more fiber, drink more water and opt for more organic foods especially green vegetables, yoghurt, garlic and onions. Olive oil, fish oils and flaxseed oil are also helpful.

But be aware that it can take several months for these measures to take effect.

Certain minerals and vitamins can also help your condition especially high doses of magnesium and vitamin B6. Folic acid is also an anti-fungal agent. Or you could try supplements such as caprylic acid, Echinacea, colloidal silver, whole leaf aloe vera juice, garlic, citrus seed extract, oatstraw tea, or probiotics such as lactobacillus acidophilus. Oil of oregano can help against skin-based fungal infections.

For women with vaginal infections it is recommended to wear cotton and non-synthetic fiber underwear, and bathing in water with essential oils such as bergamot, clary sage, lavender, ylang-ylang, clove, fennel or geranium.

Herbal Products For Candida

Acidophilus

Provides friendly bacteria which normally resides in the intestines and is often destroyed through taking prescription antibiotics, using the birth pill or steroids. It can also be depleted though a dietary shortfall. These friendly bacteria can be replaced by taking a supplement in capsule form and/or through the diet.

Antioxidants

Antioxidants protect the body against the effects of free radical damage. Well known antioxidants – beta carotene (which is converted to vitamin A by the body as it is needed), vitamin E (which works well with the antioxidant mineral selenium) and vitamin C may slow down the aging process as well as protecting the body against many different diseases.

Apple Cider Vinegar

Excellent for vaginal yeast infections and external candida conditions. It has good anti-fungal properties and can be added to warm bath water enabling a person to soak in it.

Natural Multi Vitamin & Multi Mineral Supplement

This supplements acts as an insurance policy against any shortfall of essential vitamins and minerals in the diet. If there is a shortfall, then the body will utilize the supplement. If it is not needed, then it will pass out of the body in the urine.

Caprylic Acid

Caprylic Acid is a fatty acid that is effective at killing candida yeast.

Colloidal Silver

Although not a herb, colloidal silver has many uses and has been found to be effective against many surface micro-organisms, viruses, protozoa, amoeba, fungi parasites and yeasts.

There are many different colloidal silver products on the market. You need to source one that contains 99.9 percent pure silver, without any additives.

Flaxseed Oil

Flax fibers are amongst the oldest fiber crops in the world. The use of flax for the production of linen goes back at least to ancient

Egyptian times. The flax plant has many uses. Linseed is extracted from it which is used as a dietary supplement as well as being used in various wood finishing products. It is very high in the essential fatty acids (EFAs) omega 3 and omega 6, which are essential for the prevention of onset degenerative diseases such as heart disease and stroke.

Garlic

Garlic is excellent for purging candida yeast and parasites from the body. Garlic has so many uses from using it in cooking to it being an excellent product for heart health. It also has antibacterial, antifungus and antiviral properties. Other recognized health benefits of garlic include, acting as an antibiotic and having anti-cholesterol and anti-hypertensive properties.

It is also an antioxidant which protects the body against the effects of free radical damage. Its high sulphur content assists in cell purification.

Allicin is the principle biological active compound which gives garlic its odor. Be warned. Many so called "odourless" garlic products have the active compound removed which makes it rather worthless. It can be obtained as a garlic bulb, in a capsule or in tablet form.

Grapefruit Seed Extract

Grapefruit Seed Extract is one of the most useful supplements for eliminating candida yeast. It is also an effective anti-parasitic herb which has a very bitter taste. This can be sweetened by adding a small amount of honey.

Oregano

Available in either enteric coated (meaning it will burst in the body where it is supposed to), or in liquid form, oregano possesses anti-inflammatory antiviral and anti-fungal properties which makes it especially useful for eradicating candida yeast.

Pau D' Arco

Pau D'Arco originates from Brazil and Argentina where the inner bark is used for a variety of treatments. It has excellent anti-fungal properties making it especially useful in a candida yeast program.

Peppermint Oil

Can be purchased as an enteric coated capsule or in liquid form. If liquid is used then only very tiny drops should be applied to water, otherwise it will be too strong. It is excellent for an upset stomach, to eliminate bad breath and as a general tonic.

Probiotics

Probiotics are an essential part of good health as they keep "balance" in the body, as well as aiding the digestive, intestinal and immune systems. These "friendly" bacteria produce hydrogen peroxide which kills candida; thus in addition to its other health giving benefits it is a good candida eradication supplement.

Constipation

Everyone knows what this is! Technically it's when you have "bowel movements" less than three times a week. It's something which affects twice as many women as men—four out of ten pregnant women and the elderly. Despite what some people believe, constipation doesn't lead to cancer. In the case of people with Irritable Bowel Syndrome it alternates with diarrhea.

There can be numerous reasons why you're constipated from having an overactive thyroid to lead poisoning.

When you've got acute symptoms such as rectal bleeding, abdominal pain and cramps, nausea and vomiting and involuntary loss of weight, it's time to see your doctor.

Doctors will assess your diet, examine you physically and maybe try blood tests, an abdominal X-ray and/or a Barium enema.

What Can I Do?

Basically drink more water and improve your diet by eating more organic fruits and vegetables, but especially put more fiber in your diet.

Exercise is also an important part of good colon health. If you lead a sedentary lifestyle then consider an exercise program that you would enjoy doing, otherwise you will soon get bored with it and give us.

Why not join a gym where a qualified instructor will work out a program for you? Alternatively go bike riding, play tennis, do work in the garden or a 30 minute brisk walk five days each week. All these will work wonders for your colon health, in addition to supporting all your body systems.

Sometimes laxatives are necessary—but should only be used with caution. Long term use can lead to a "lazy" colon which will make matters worse.

Herbal Products For Constipation

Cascara Sagrada

Well known for its quick acting laxative effects. It is often used for constipation in addition to helping purge toxins from the body. It promotes peristaltic action—the movement of waste matter through the colon, and stimulates secretions from the gall bladder, liver, pancreas and stomach.

Guar Gum

Is often used in fiber blends as it provides soluble digestible fiber. The body needs non-soluble as well as soluble fiber. Guar gum soaks toxins up like a sponge, has a laxative effect, curbs appetite and is beneficial in lowering cholesterol.

Psyllium

An excellent source of dietary fiber. Psyllium is gluten free and is therefore a useful fiber source for those suffering from celiac disease or gluten intolerance.

It expands dramatically from the size of the original seeds and it is therefore essential to drink plenty of water with this product.

Psyllium absorbs toxins from the intestinal tract and binds them to fecal matter for elimination.

As it is a bulking agent, it often gives a feeling of fullness and discourages a person from over eating.

Detoxing With A Herbal Colon Cleanse

Your body is a wonderful machine—think of it like a car engine. Over time your car's engine gets sluggish so you take it to a repair shop to get it serviced. The engine oil is changed and so is the filter, in addition, other items may need attention too. When the car is returned, there is a noticeable difference. It runs smoother and has more power.

The human body is just the same. Over time it get sluggish, and various symptoms may arise, such as headaches, lack of energy, lack of appetite or possibly skin disorders. What your body is telling you is that it is time for some attention. And this is where detoxing often comes in.

But before we talk about detoxing, a quick word about toxins. What are they? Toxins take two forms (external and internal) and impact various parts of the body.

The external part comprises what we breathe in and what we eat and drink—usually a Western diet which is high in fats, sugars and chemicals and low in fiber. Other factors include: a lack of exercise, constipation, use of various medications as well as other lifestyle choices.

The internal part comprises the metabolic by-product of the diet. When the body digests food it creates toxic wastes. When the body is in healing and repairing mode it creates toxic wastes. If you experience negative emotions like anger and stress the body will create toxins.

These poisons build up in the colon, liver, kidneys and blood, in addition to causing inflammation in joint tissue which can lead to arthritis. Usually the early visible sign of toxins is when an eruption occurs on the surface of the skin. This can be in the form of pimples, blackheads, puss spots and other skin conditions.

Longer term, major health issues could arise such as chronic fatigue, depression, diabetes, heart, kidney and liver disease or cancer. Premature aging could also be a concern.

All these toxic factors impact the immune system which is the body's protection mechanism against disease. When the immune system is not working properly, it is then unable to protect the body against airborne invaders which enter through the nose, mouth and skin as well as metabolic changes within the body's structure.

The colon is one of the major areas where toxins reside. This is in the form of impacted fecal matter which may have been there for many years. It become a breeding ground for all kinds of unfriendly bacteria, parasites, worms and amoeba like structures all of which have one purpose—to do your body harm. They are not your friends.

Many people who undertake a colon cleanse often lose as much as 7 to 9 pounds in body weight. This is all impacted toxic matter that has been purged out of the system, along with any parasites that reside there.

Herbs are one of the best natural ways to undertake a colon cleanse. I have included a list at the end of this section. But briefly, herbs such as licorice root, milk thistle, horsetail, violet leaf and passionflower root as well as a fiber source such as psyllium are often used.

When undertaking a detoxing program it is important to drink plenty of filtered water to assist the liver in eliminating toxins from your body. Notice I mentioned filtered water, or if this is not possible then the best quality water you can find.

Do not use tap water. This is full of chemicals and is not good for you. It will not be very beneficial in a detoxing program. Chlorine and fluoride are often added to tap water in many states or districts and countries.

Fluoride is a by-product of aluminium processing and is highly toxic and poisonous. The aluminium industry had to dispose of this waste somehow, so they did a good "selling job" by convincing everyone that this poisonous and toxic substance was good for dental health amongst other things.

The trouble is this toxic substance ends up in the liver and kidneys and other organs where it resides in a toxic form until it is removed with a detoxing program.

Everyone reacts to a detox in different ways. You could experience symptoms such as headaches, a sore throat, muscle aches, constipation or flu-like symptoms. These conditions are only temporary and this is the body's way of telling you that the program is working and that internal adjustments are being made.

Following on from your detox program, you should consider making some dietary adjustments, by only eating organic produce: meat, poultry, vegetables and fruits, as well as oily fish (mackerel, tuna, salmon); fish should preferably be grilled or poached, not fried.

Increase your fiber intake. Remember fiber is one of the best forms of absorbing toxins. Psyllium in particular acts like a sponge in absorbing toxins and eliminating them along with fecal matter.

Don't forget whole grains, nuts and seeds which are a good source of fiber and contain beneficial oils in addition to vitamins and minerals.

Getting adequate sleep and rest—which allows the body to repair and rejuvenate itself—as well as introducing an exercise program if you don't have one already will be beneficial to all your body systems, but especially the circulatory system.

One final thing. Always consult your doctor or a qualified naturopathic doctor (ND) before starting any detox program or making dietary changes. It might be that you have health issues which could make a detox program or dietary changes unsuitable for you. So take appropriate advice beforehand.

Herbal Products For Detoxing

This is rather a long list. You may be well informed and able to make your own selection. If you are unsure, then you may wish to discuss this list with a naturopathic doctor (ND) or other qualified natural health care provider.

Diuretic and Laxative Herbs

Alfalfa

Alfalfa is a grass which contains all the essential amino acids as well as being rich in trace minerals and enzymes. It is frequently taken to lessen the effects of hay fever allergies. It is also fed to horses as a counter to arthritic conditions and digestive problems.

As it is a good source of fiber, it is useful for detoxifying the body in addition to improving liver health.

Cascara Sagrada

Well known for it quick acting laxative effects. It is often used for constipation in addition to helping purge toxins from the body. It promotes peristaltic action—the movement of waste matter through the colon, and stimulates secretions from the gall bladder, liver, pancreas and stomach.

Guar Gum

Is often used in fiber blends as it provides soluble digestible fiber. The body needs non-soluble as well as soluble fiber. Guar gum soaks toxins up like a sponge, has a laxative effect, curbs appetite and is beneficial in lowering cholesterol.

Hibiscus Flower

Hibiscus flower have anti-bacterial properties as well as being an anti-parasitic. In addition it acts as a diuretic and is soothing.

Licorice Root

Licorice root provides nutritional support to the adrenal glands which is especially important when the body is under stress.

It boosts energy in addition to supporting the digestive system. It is usually added to Chinese formulas in order to bring balance and harmony to the ingredients.

In a detoxing program it will rid the body of over 1,200 toxins without any side effects. Licorice root is very sweet and is a great addition to herbal teas.

It helps regulate blood sugar levels and assists in neutralizing the effects of hypoglycemia; licorice also helps soothe any irritation in mucus membranes.

Finally, it relaxes muscles and is a natural muscle builder and strengthener.

Marshmallow Root

Marshmallow is a mild laxative as well as a diuretic. Its mucilaginous content provides relief for an irritated digestive tract as well as providing moisture to dry tissues.

Psyllium

An excellent source of dietary fiber. Psyllium is gluten free and is therefore a useful fiber source for those suffering from celiac disease or gluten intolerance.

It expands dramatically from the size of the original seeds and it is therefore essential to drink plenty of water with this product.

Psyllium absorbs toxins from the intestinal tract and binds them to fecal matter for elimination.

As it is a bulking agent, it often gives a feeling of fullness and discourages a person from over eating.

Violet Leaf

Is a good source of vitamin C and beta carotene (which the body converts to vitamin A as needed). Violet leaf has antifungal properties in addition to being a diuretic and laxative.

Yucca Root

Yucca root is high in fiber content and as such, is an excellent herb for digestive and intestinal problems. It can rid the body of undigested waste toxins which reside in the colon and cause foul smelling gasses.

Historically, yucca root has been used as an anti-inflammatory and laxative agent that purges toxins from joints which if left untreated, can cause inflammation that then leads to joint problems such as arthritis. Yucca is also effective at eliminating toxins from the blood, kidneys, liver and lymph.

Liver Support Herbs

Cascara Sagrada

Well known for it quick acting laxative effects. It is often used for constipation in addition to helping purge toxins from the body. It promotes peristaltic action—the movement of waste matter through the colon, and stimulates secretions from the gall bladder, liver, pancreas and stomach.

Dandelion

Dandelion has been used for centuries to stimulate the liver to detoxify poisons. It is important for promoting good circulatory system function and strengthening weak arteries.

Milk Thistle

One of the compounds in milk thistle—silymarin promotes the elimination of toxins from the liver. Milk thistle also protects the liver from the effects of substance abuse and alcohol consumption. It has anti-inflammatory properties to protect the liver from stress and injury.

Parasite Expulsion Herbs

Black Walnut

Black walnut is an excellent anti-parasitic herb, especially against worms. It also has a high iodine content, which is good for energy as it supports thyroid function.

Garlic

Garlic is excellent for purging candida yeast and parasites from the body. Garlic has so many uses from using it in cooking to it being an excellent product for heart health. It also has antibacterial, antifungus and antiviral properties. Other recognized health benefits of garlic include, acting as an antibiotic and having anti-cholesterol and anti-hypertensive properties.

It is also an antioxidant which protects the body against the effects of free radical damage. Its high sulphur content assists in cell purification.

Allicin is the principle biological active compound which gives garlic its odor. Be warned. Many so called "odourless" garlic products have the active compound removed which makes it rather worthless. It can be obtained as a garlic bulb, in a capsule or in tablet form.

Pumpkin Seeds

One of the best tasting of all the anti-parasite herbal products. The seeds can be eaten as a snack. In fact they taste so good that you cannot eat enough of them. Pumpkin seeds are very effective against tapeworms as well as other types of parasites. They also serve as a good source of linolenic acid—one of the essential fatty acids (EFAs) which are essential for good health.

Herbs to Soothe an Irritated Digestive System and Urinary Tract

Cranberry

Cranberry's main purpose is to treat bacterial infections in the bladder. It is often combined with buchu herb.

Irish Moss

Irish moss is a type of seaweed that soothes an irritated gastrointestinal tract. It is also used in hand and body lotion products to alleviate various skin conditions.

Passionflower

A natural sedative, passionflower will help you sleep without leaving a groggy feeling the next morning. It is beneficial for calming the nervous system, and stress conditions.

Passionflower slows the breakdown of neurotransmitters which pass chemical messages between the body's cells, as well as working with certain enzymes. It also assists in calming an irritable bowel, as well as killing certain bacteria.

Herbs that have Antioxidant, Antiseptic and Anti-Inflammatory Properties

Capsicum

Also called cayenne pepper, this is the body's disinfectant. It helps rebuild tissue in the stomach as well as assisting in healing stomach and intestinal ulcers.

Capsicum has antioxidant and antiseptic properties in addition to providing support to the circulatory system. Its catalytic action helps in the transmission of other herbs to parts of the body where they are needed.

Chickweed

Chickweed is used to strengthen the colon and stomach as well as helping to dissolve plaque and fatty deposits. Chickweed has healing properties for stomach ulcers and inflammation in the colon.

Cranberry

Cranberry's main purpose is to treat bacterial infections in the bladder. It is often combined with buchu herb.

Gentian Root

Gentian root helps in the breakdown of fats and proteins and assists in the body's assimilation of iron and vitamin B12. As it has a cooling effect on body tissue, this helps reduce infections and inflammation. Gentian root also promotes digestive secretions.

Witch Hazel

Witch hazel has excellent anti-inflammatory and antiseptic properties. As it has a high flavonoid content, this helps to heal damaged blood vessels.

Herbs that Act as Blood Purifiers, Diuretics and Energy Providers

Burdock Root

Burdock root is one of the best blood purifiers to clear circulatory and lymphatic congestion. As it assists in alleviating excess body fluids, toxins are more easily purged from the body.

Other uses for burdock root: aids in reducing swelling around joints, expels surplus calcium deposits and cleanses the blood of harmful acids.

Chlorella

Chlorella contains over 19 amino acids of these eight are the essential ones in addition to beta carotene (which the body converts to vitamin A as needed), potassium and other important vitamins and minerals, plus enzymes.

Chlorella has natural antioxidant properties and as such, is a good detoxifier, cell enhancer and blood cleanser.

When taken as a liquid it eliminates body odors from the digestive tract, and is also an excellent mouth wash to eliminate bad breath.

Echinacea

There are various strains of Echinacea. It is used to support the immune system and is involved in the production of white blood cells, which assists the body in fight infection. Echinacea purges toxins from the blood and enhances lymphatic drainage.

Fennel Seed

Fennel seed has several uses including: supporting the digestive and nervous systems, alleviating the effects of colic, gas and intestinal problems. It also has diuretic properties.

Fenugreek

Fenugreek is a respiratory system herb which assists in expelling mucous, phlegm and infections from the lungs, and toxic waste through the lymphatic system. In addition, fenugreek is able to dissolve a hardened build up of mucous which can then be eliminated.

Garlic

Garlic is excellent for purging candida yeast and parasites from the body. Garlic has so many uses from using it in cooking to it being an excellent product for heart health. It also has antibacterial, anti-fungus and antiviral properties. Other recognized health benefits of garlic include, acting as an antibiotic and having anti-cholesterol and anti-hypertensive properties.

It is also an antioxidant which protects the body against the effects of free radical damage. Its high sulphur content assists in cell purification.

Allicin is the principle biological active compound which gives garlic its odor. Be warned. Many so called "odourless" garlic products have the active compound removed which makes it rather worthless. It can be obtained as a garlic bulb, in a capsule or in tablet form.

Ginger

In India's Ayurvedic medicine ginger is called vishwabhesaj "the universal medicine". The pungent and warming properties of ginger have long been used to enhance the "fire" in the body, which is responsible for proper digestion, body heat, visual perception, hunger, thirst, the luster of the skin, the light in the eyes, the clarity in the mind, intelligence, determination and courage.

Ginger is an excellent cleansing agent for the colon, skin and kidneys. Provides support to the respiratory system. It is often used to alleviate the effects of a cold or flu. Many people take it as a natural alternative for motion and morning sickness.

Horsetail

Horsetail is one of the best herbs for improving digestion as well as relieving symptoms of bloating and gas.

As it is rich in trace minerals, it is an excellent herb for assisting the healing of the skin, bones and cartilage. As it is also an antifungal agent and diuretic it is a good herb in a detoxing program.

Mullein

A mucilaginous herb which soothes irritated tissue. It is very beneficial for respiratory system health.

Oatstraw

Oatstraw is a good source of minerals for nourishing bones, hair, skin and nails.

It helps calm the nervous system and can assist in cases of depression and exhaustion.

Slippery Elm

Slippery elm is very soothing to inflamed tissue—especially in the gastrointestinal tract—and as a result, is excellent for tissue healing. It is easily digested and has good laxative properties.

Skin Cleansing Herbs

Burdock Root

Burdock root is one of the best blood purifiers to clear circulatory and lymphatic congestion. As it assists in alleviating excess body fluids, toxins are more easily purged from the body.

Other uses for burdock root: aids in reducing swelling around joints, expels surplus calcium deposits and cleanses the blood of harmful acids.

Capsicum

Also called cayenne pepper is the body's disinfectant. It helps rebuild tissue in the stomach as well as assisting in healing stomach and intestinal ulcers.

Capsicum has antioxidant and antiseptic properties in addition to providing support to the circulatory system. Its catalytic action helps in the transmission of other herbs to parts of the body where they are needed.

Colloidal Silver

This is available as a liquid or in gel form. Colloidal silver has been used for centuries to treat all manner of body conditions. It is especially useful for skin problems whether acquired through an injury or an infection. The gel makes a good general skin cleanser.

Ginger

Ginger is an excellent cleansing agent for the colon, skin and kidneys. Provides support to the respiratory system. It is often used to alleviate the effects of a cold or flu. Many people take it as a natural alternative for motion and morning sickness.

Oregano

Available in either enteric coated (meaning it will burst in the body where it is supposed to), or in liquid form, oregano possesses anti-inflammatory antiviral and anti-fungal properties and is an excellent herb for protecting the skin.

Peppermint Oil

Can be purchased as an enteric coated capsule or in liquid form. If liquid is used then only very tiny drops should be applied to water, otherwise it will be too strong. It is excellent for an upset stomach, to eliminate bad breath and as a general tonic.

Yellow Dock

Assists with elimination and is one of the best blood builders in the herbal arsenal.

To Sum Up

Remember that parasites and worms will harm your body and rob it of essential nutrients, which can cause disease and illness. We can't actually see many of these malignant microbes which invade us. But that doesn't mean they're not there. We should realise that our body is a battleground—and like all good military commanders we have to deploy all the means at our disposal to fend them off.

Many people have yeast infections, but unless they get out of control then they can be left alone. It is when the body gets out of balance that remedial action needs to be taken. Otherwise more serious health issues can arise.

Constipation is a major consequence of a Western diet which is high in fats, sugar, salt, additives and colors, and low in fiber.

Then add in the busy lifestyle that many people lead where there is no time to sit down and eat a meal properly, in addition to a lack of exercise; all this adds up to an unbalanced body and often constipation is a consequence of this.

I sometimes think that the Spanish and Italians have the right idea. Over the years I have worked in both these countries, and it is not unusual for lunch to take several hours. Lunchtime siesta is the order of the day, where people relax, take their time eating their food, enjoy a glass of wine and enjoy good conversation.

Contrast this with what I often see in the US where buying lunch from a drive-thru is quite common, then the recipient eats lunch whilst driving to their next appointment, or alternatively, I often see people eating lunch whilst walking down the street. Not relaxing to eat properly puts the body under tremendous stress. No wonder there are so many cases of indigestion, heartburn, ulcers and overweight to name a few.

Finally, detoxing the body is all important to purge the body of poisonous toxins, which if left untreated, can have a major long term effect on a person's health.

It is a good idea to undertake a cleansing program in the spring and fall, or every six months. You will be amazed at how much better you will feel afterwards.

Remember though to consult your doctor or a qualified naturopathic doctor (ND) before undertaking a parasite program, candida program, alleviating the effects of constipation, doing a body detox or changing your diet.

This is especially important if you have any medical condition which you are undergoing treatment for.

Notice To My Readers

Some of the herbal products mentioned in this book may not be available in your country due to misguided government regulatory reasons, or an attempt by regulatory agencies to deny your choice of using "natural" products as opposed to drug based medications.

If this applies to your country, then you can always try the Internet. In this enlightened age of global communications, at the touch of a button, with a little effort on your part, you can often find the products that you require, and most suppliers will ship their products globally.

About The Author

Brian B Jacques has been a natural health researcher for over thirty years. He has presented seminars worldwide on such diverse subjects as Health Related issues, Motivation and Personal Development. In addition he has written numerous eBooks, newsletters and articles on these subjects.

His very popular Series of Mini-Health Books includes:

- An Easy Way To Understand Eczema and Psoriasis
- An Easy Way To Understand Stress and Depression
- Amino Acids & Enzymes—What Are They & Why Do You Need Them
- An Easy Way To Understand Vitamins and Minerals
- An Easy Way To Understand Crohn's Disease and IBD
- An Easy Way To Understand Body Building For Men And Women
- An Easy Way To Understand Alzheimer's Disease
- An Easy Way To Understand Herpes
- An Easy Way To Understand Parkinson's Disease
- An Easy Way To Understand Autism
- An Easy Way To Understand Fibromyalgia
- The Little A–Z Dictionary of Herbal Remedies
- Effective Methods To Stop Smoking
- The Magic Of Vitamins & Minerals
- An Easy Way To Understand Your Body Systems
- An Easy Way To Understand Erectile Dysfunction
- An Easy Way To Understand Heart Disease, High Blood Pressure & Stroke
- An Easy Way To Understand Detoxing For Men & Women
- How To Lose Weight After 40
- How To Lose Weight And Maintain Your Ideal Weight Permanently

Another thirty titles in the Mini-Health Series are currently in preparation.

All these books are available as Kindle Editions (available from the Kindle Store on Amazon.com, and other countries Amazon sites where the Kindle platform is supported.) Many of these books are also available for the Barnes and Noble "Nook".

In addition, all these titles will shortly be available as print editions from the Amazon website.

Made in the USA
Charleston, SC
19 September 2014